Carb Cycling

Proven Carb Cycling Weight Loss Strategies. (Includes the Easiest Carb Cycling Plan in The World)

By Richard Huntley

Table of Contents

How to achieve your goals...

Success with carb cycling...

Conclusion

Introduction

I want to thank you and congratulate you for reading this book on carb cycling and I'm excited to share with you a lot of these breakthrough strategies.

This book contains proven steps and strategies on how to carb cycle for weight loss.

Here's the most important thing you will learn inside this brand-new carb cycling book. Until you discover exactly how you can still eat high carb foods the right way, you'll never really learn how to burn off stubborn belly fat once and for all.

So you might be thinking what's the big secret that keeps the world-class fitness professionals and the countries that have the lowest obesity rate in the world such as Japan so lean and healthy year after year?

Simple... it is carb cycling.

And the great news is this isn't some elite strategy only reserved for people such as competitive athletes you might see on TV or fitness models with superior genetics.

You can really use the exact same techniques to produce real amazing results for yourself.

Just before we dive into my top carb cycling strategies that me tell you a little about myself.

Hi, my name is Richard Huntley and I am the founder of RH Martial Fitness, and over the past 7 years I've been helping the "everyday person" all over the world learn the truth about how to lose weight without crazy yo-yo dieting or doing hours of endless boring cardio.

Every month I help over 300,000 folks through the power of the internet, whether it's a busy stay at home mum juggling family commitments, to guys and gals who have busy jobs and there lifestyle won't let them have the time to train like an athlete.

I say this because back in 2007 I was actually an athlete myself in the martial arts, and got the chance to represent my country of Great Britain.

I had to get in fantastic shape for my competitions and that's when I discovered a whole lot more about weight loss and workouts by learning from some of the best mentors and coaches around the world.

Now it's my time to share my knowledge with and you're going to love this book on the amazing benefits of carb cyling.

Why Carb Cycling Works

In this first chapter we are going to look at how the Japanese are some of the healthiest and leanest people in the world and how you can adapt your current diet to using these principles in your everyday life and get fit, healthy and lean.

The funny thing is did you know the Japanese are some of leanest and healthiest people on the entire planet? I know when I travel many times to train with some of the top Japanese martial art masters i really got into understanding how their culture works along with their lifestyle approach to eating and exercising.

Many people are surprised when I tell them they are more likely to reach 100 years old than anyone else in the world, and in fact most of the researchers tend to continue studying and looking into their diets for the last 100 years. It's even been known that some people call their home the land of immortals.

In addition to not only their long life's expectancy, they are known for their unusually low rate of cardiovascular disease and even types of certain cancers. They are actually less likely to die from heart disease, and seven times less likely to die from prostate cancer.

This is all compared to the average Western person. Now I'm as patriotic and proud as any other Western person for their country but I still understand that their needs to be changes within the diet industry and that's why I'm continuing to reveal the truth about how to keep fit and healthy with happiness and longevity.

The Carb Cycle Lifestyle

Now just like the Japanese I'm going to show you how you can still eat high-carbohydrate meals and lose weight without the fuss of yo-yo dieting or grueling cardio exercise workouts for hours every day. Let's face it; it's not much of a fun life to live if you've been told by a fitness magazine to work out for hours all the time restrict yourself daily with certain fad diets.

Especially if you are the everyday person with a busy lifestyle and family to take care of and need to.

Now in order to burn stomach fat and lose weight, we've been told to just eat less carbs and exercise more. And you could put this in other words which could be seen as putting your body in a calorie deficit to burn off more than you take in.

Now we all know this come work but it's temporarily.

And that's exactly why 95% of the population gains all if not more of their weight back on within the first year of starting their low carb crash diet or as he seen in the 1990s the popular low-fat diet.

But here's the thing to remember. Do you really think lean and healthy people just like the Japanese obsess over choosing specific low glycaemic foods or counting calories all the time? I can tell you from first-hand experience they don't, and you do not need to either.

If you enjoy counting calories I say stick with it. But the average guy and ladies I meet in the real world really don't enjoy doing it.

The lean people simply focus on the foods whether they are a high carb food or low carb food that burn fat the most and keep their bodies healthy long-term.

It always comes down to the quality of the food you are eating first.

Living Lean

In order to boost your metabolism, you will understand that hormones will play a big part of the fat burning process. I've seen people obsess too much on the low carb side of things and the big problem is sometimes it leads to a thing called metabolic damage and in the long run this can really mess up your body's hormones and make it very tough to get your body back to where you want it to be.

What are the benefits of carb cycling?

- **You'll still eat the foods you love**

- **You'll feel better overall and have more energy**

- **You can maintain and build healthy lean muscle**

- **You'll learn how to shed off your access weight and body fat**

- **It really fits any type of lifestyle**

How Carb Cycling Can Work For You

Really a carb cycling diet is a nutritional method approach that varies between periods of high carbohydrate intake and a low carbohydrate intake. Obviously carb cycling diets really focus on your carbohydrate intake due to its most important role with the fat burning hormones such as insulin and other metabolic processes that are related for you to lose body fat and gain lean muscle.

When it comes down to the primary purpose of carb cycling it is really to deplete and refill your muscle glycogen stores that helps us regulate our fat burning hormones to keep us in what we call fat burning mode, so you are literally a fat burning machine 24 seven. Good times!

A higher carbohydrate intake causes stimulation and the main release of insulin in the blood, which helps grab hold of nutrients and shuttle them straight into your muscles out which replenishes lost muscle glycogen from doing your specific workouts. Also high-carbohydrate days can top up your energy levels and prepare your body for some intense training days ahead which is why you see athletes vary their carbohydrate levels from day-to-day.

Looking at now the lower carbohydrate days, these are the days that promote fat metabolism in which causes your body to switch from carbohydrates to fat for its main fuel source. Now specifically on your lower carbohydrate days you will burn through the glycogen you have stored from your higher carbohydrate days and after that tap Straight in to your fat stores for energy.

This overall process can help keep your body become more receptive to your fat burning hormone with a better insulin response, which in doing so improves fuel source efficiency to your muscles which will help you perform a better workout overall.

How to Setup Your Carb Cycling Diet

Now there are many ways to set up your carb cycling diet. One way you can do it is by aligning high and low carb days with your workouts. On the days you workout harder you can have yourself a higher carbohydrate day.

On the days you're performing a lighter cardio style exercise stick to a low carbohydrate intake. A lot of people aim for round three high carb days and four low carb days but really it depends on your workout schedule and your sensitivity to eating carbohydrates.

If you're getting ready for a holiday or vacation or special event I would recommend having more low carb days, and keeping down the high carb days as we will want to target body fat to look sharp and lean for a special occasion.

How many carbohydrates?

On average we see that low carbohydrate days people carb cycling tends to aim for around the 50 g mark. Doing this will allow the body to effectively use up existing glycogen stores and switch over to using fat as fuel. At around 50 g you can ensure that you're sparing less lean muscle protein from being used as fuel.

On high-carbohydrate days on average, you can look up and vary from anywhere at 200 g plus but again let me help you understand that the amounts really all depends on your response to carbohydrates and how efficiently use up the carbs once you put them into your body every day.

To be honest at the start you are better off sticking to the lower side of the scale with your carbohydrate intake for both high days and low days and working from there.

Three nutrients you need to keep an eye on!

Protein. Overall protein builds and maintains muscles and most importantly how muscles burn calories like wildfire. Protein also breaks down more slowly than carbs and fat, but most of all especially if you're looking for weight loss as a protein rich meal will help you keep full for longer so you won't be snacking throughout the day. That's why I always recommend people start their day with a good source of protein and fats.

Carbs. As discussed already earlier carbohydrates are the preferred fuel source for your muscles and organs and they come in healthy versions such as vegetables, fruits, and some grains plus legumes. The not so healthy versions are things like cakes, cookies, doughnuts, sodas and many more fast absorbing carbohydrates that are just full of junk and chemicals that clog up our bodies and riddle them with disease and fat storage over time.

Healthy carbs are really crucial for burning your calories and since they break down more slowly, and these healthy carbohydrates keep your blood sugar and energy levels steady throughout the day and they keep you burning calories throughout the day which is obviously what you want if you're here to lose weight.

Healthy fats. Here's the real deal with eating fats. Lots of people over the past years have been afraid of eating them and there really is no problem with eating certain fats, but the main problem that people run into is having highly processed fats (trans fats) and this causes their diets to also have a higher omega six intake rather than having a good balance of omega threes to Omega sixes.

Foods such as oily fish have a great number of omega threes which can help balance out your daily intake of omega threes to Omega six. With this you will not cause the body to have an imbalance of bad inflammation.

These types of healthy fats when consumed will definitely help your brain function better and prevent heart disease, stroke, arthritis and even from depression. Like I mentioned before with proteins for breakfast healthy fats are also essential to help keep your energy levels steady and keep you from feeling hungry which in the end makes you not snack out on junk throughout the day.

The Truth About Fiber

I'm sure you've heard by now within the health and fitness industry that you should always choose to eat good fibrous starchy carbs instead of pure white starches if your goal is to lose body fat.

The most popular example with this could be replacing white rice with brown rice because Brown Rice has more fiber. Now the main difference between white and brown rice is processing and nutritional content, with only one layer which is the outermost being removed when producing the brown rice.

When white rice is produced everything gets removed which only leaves the starchy main component of the grain. This means pretty much all of the key vitamins and minerals in white rice are lost including fiber. Now you can really see why we've been told to use brown rice instead of consuming white rice. If you are trying to eat healthy balanced meals and keep your blood sugar stable throughout the day and especially if you are a prolific exerciser this can be a good choice for some people.

But each cup of brown rice contains only 3.5 g of fiber which is for every 45 g of complex carbs. This would mean he would be looking at five whole cups of brown rice just to get her of your daily fiber intake.

Now you can see why trying to get more fiber from starches can sometimes be a waste of time and really could be making you fat if you do not go careful with this approach that the weight loss industry and fitness gurus have been telling us.

The small amount of fiber you will get from this can be a nice bonus, but it's not really what's going to make a big impact on your weight loss. It's another food myth, and you should be easily getting enough fiber throughout your daily basis with your intake of fibrous fruits and vegetables.

So the real take-home point with this is to consume starches with your metabolic needs and not just because they have a little bit of fiber within them. So like I've mentioned before save your starchy carbohydrates to fuel your high intensity activity days or to recover faster from your workouts and keep your metabolic rates at a healthy level. Another key point is to always combine them with a complete protein and vegetables whenever possible, as this will prevent unhealthy blood sugar spikes and help keep your body in fat burning mode.

Cheat Day on Carb Cycling Diet?

The thing is, one of the main benefit's of carb cycling is your cravings for junk foods tend to decrease. So yes cheat days tend to be higher carbohydrate days but a lot of people tend to go off track and eat too many junk loaded with bad sugars and fats that result you with unnecessary weight gain.

So if you really do want to have a cheat day in the week, you can by all means as it's your body and it's up to you but I would really looking to still eating as clean as possible throughout most of your cheat day.

How Long to Keep Carb Cycling?

There really is no specific reason you have stop your carb cycling style diet, as it's easy to maintain and because you're always cycling your macronutrients your body does not plateau as much compared to other dieting strategies.

I would say to at least test trial yourself with the carb cycling strategy for six weeks and see how your body responds and how you look and feel. Having this diet strategy along with a great workout plan will definitely get you some results if you have the right mindset and are ready to take massive action and not give up as there will be some days that will be more challenging than others.

A Schedule for Carb Cycling

Now there really is not just "one way" to carb cycle but below I'll share with you a typical carb cycling week to help you maintain your fat loss results week after week if you are looking to lose some serious pounds.

Monday, low carb day

Tuesday, low carb day

Wednesday, high carb day

Thursday, low carb day

Friday, high carb day

Saturday, low carb day

Sunday, high carb day

Now like I mentioned before everybody has different goals and everybody's body will respond differently to each other we are all individuals in this world. With this being said this is all about testing to see what works for you and if you need to cut out one of those high carb days, I would say do so, or if this schedule hits the sweet spot for you and it works like a charm simply stick to it.

The Easiest Carb Cycling Plan in the World!

These rules I'm about to share with you on carb cycling is extremely simple but effective.

Step one. On days you do high intensity activities or lift weights, eat your starchy carbs along with healthy proteins, vegetables, and healthy fats.

Step two. On the day you are either not working out or you are doing a low intensity style workout such as going for a 30 min walk to listen to an audio book or walk your dog like I do, you will want to not eat any starchy carbs but still continuing with eating your good sources of protein, vegetables, and specific healthy fats.

Some Good Healthy Nutrient Carbs for you

White or sweet potato

Oatmeal

Quinoa

Buckwheat pasta

Fruits, berries are best

Rice

Some Junk Carbs for you to Avoid

Muffins

Pizza

Cakes, cookies or other desserts

Doughnuts

Any sugar packed processed foods

Sample high carb day meal plan

Breakfast

Oatmeal, first cup of oats with berries and a few walnuts

Snack

Handful of almonds

Lunch

a whole wheat tortilla wrap with chicken, salsa, and lettuce.

Optional two snack

An Apple or banana

Dinner

Whole-grain pitta, chopped tomatoes, mozzarella, Basil. Cook in oven like normal pizza.

Sample Low carb day meal plan

Breakfast:

3-4 whole eggs (scrambled, poached, or fried)

Add in some fiber veggies like broccoli.

Snack:

Handful of almonds

Lunch at Restaurant:

Salad with lots of meat and vegetables

Optional two Snack:

Handful of almonds

Dinner at Home:

Grass fed beef burger wrapped in lettuce with salad

Quick cheat tip

You will notice on both high carb days and low carb days they are virtually the same with including lots of protein vegetables and fats. I only major difference is that we swap the grains and starches for veggies.

2 Main Carb Cycling Questions Answered...

How many carbs should I eat in every meal?

I wouldn't worry too much about counting grams of carbs. But I have wrote general rule within this book.

An easier way to remember is that on your high activity days you up your carb intake and on your low activity days decrease your carb intake.

What if I tend to get hungry on the lower carb days?

It may well happen that you tend to get hungry on your low carb days, this is because you are avoiding certain starchy carbohydrates and maybe you were used to consuming lots of fast absorbing carbs before.

Either way the best approach for you to go by is to add more protein and healthy fats plus vegetables to your meals.

How to achieve your goals...

Here's the real truth, and if you can get one simple life lesson from me to you inside this book, it would be that the only person who is responsible for your success with achieving your health and life style goals are you.

Really that should excite you because you have the key towards your destiny, and even though it may sound a little scary because we don't exactly know what will happen in the future, you can still steer it towards the direction you really want if you take responsibility starting today.

Remember i can help guide you and teach you the strategies that will take your body to its true level of potential but you are the only one that can actually do it.

You are in the driver's seat. It's how you response to life's challenges that will make the biggest impact on the areas you wish to improve.

The main problem is it's not easy. If it were, everyone would be walking around with a million dollar figure that they would be proud of.

A lot of us pull ourselves into the blame game when times get tough and we are unhappy with something. I want you to switch this around and always look at yourself rather than others.

Could you imagine what would happen if more people started doing this? Yes there would be a whole lot less conflicts in the world. Rather than run others down, i do my best you lift others up, and this way you'll have a far better feeling of compassion and fulfillment in life.

You may be thinking, wait Rich... what has all this got to do with carb cycling? My response is an easy one... Everything!

You see, everything starts within the mind and also with a body connection, and if you can get that right with a strong, focused and determined mindset, it makes things like carb cycling and others strategies a lot easier to implement.

Create New Habits

99% of all failures come from people who have a habit of making excuses.

If you are going to want to take your body from where it is now to the best shape of your life both mentally and physically, you're going to have to give up all your excuses, and all the victim stories, and all the reasons why you can't do something.

So let's start fresh, it doesn't matter about your past failures, and i'm not so interested in them to be honest. All i care about is where you are heading and how you feel right now. This is all you should be putting your focus on too.

Have you ever heard the saying, if you keep on doing what you've always done, you'll keep on getting what you've always got.

If you keep up with the old past habits and expect different results to happen, you will be bitterly disappointed. The day you make a change is the day your body and lifestyle begins to get better!

It's simple...

The bottom line is that you are the one who is creating your life the way it is. The life and results whether you are unhappy with your bodyweight, or lack energy and always feel lethargic throughout the day, it is all the result of your past actions.

You are in charge of what you say and what you do. You are in charge of your own mindset and the choices you want to make.

The good news is that i can already see if you are reading this book that you are ready to make the change in your life. Most folks will moan about how it's bad for them and they hate the way their body looks and feels but will do nothing about it.

You are different. Deep down i know you have the power to achieve anything you want.

Pay attention to this...

Once you begin implementing your new diet and workout strategies that you learn from various sources, you will understand that most important thing once you get started.

Results don't lie.

The fastest way to success with achieving your body transformation goals will be finding what's working for you and what so much isn't. You will find that you are either getting closer towards your goals or you are not.

Obviously at this point you will want to look at what's working for you and why. This pattern will show what works best for you.

So if we take the amount of carbs you are consuming throughout your week days both on high days and low days, you will find the sweet spot for you. You'll feel better overall throughout the day and you will smash through your workouts feeling energized and setting new personal bests.

If you are looking to drop some extra pounds of stubborn body fat you'll also see that when you test and find the sweet spot with eating certain foods the excess weight will drop off.

Now where some people get a little frustrated is when nothing happens right away. But when you do find the perfect point for both workouts and nutrition you'll be on to a winning streak and in what i call peak performance.

So start to keep a weekly journal and track what you are doing so this way when you do have some success, you can see exactly how you did it. The good news is that some people will take what i have said in this book and take action on the strategies immediately and see the results come in week after week.

I know this because when i work closely with private coaching client's who have used similar strategies to the carb cycling ones inside this book and in the past they have seen these kind of speedy results too.

Success with carb cycling...

Be 100% clear with yourself before you take action.

Some of the best advice i ever had was to write down your reason "why" you want to achieve your goal. So as we are on the topic of carb cycling, i could ask you why do you want to carb cycle? What's the reason why?

Now it could be for a number of reasons and that's your unique reason. But a common one i see is because the person wants to lose weight... This ok but i would still like to dive a little deeper.

So get out your piece of paper and a pen and start your writing for why you want to achieve your goals. If we dive a little deeper than just because "i want to lose weight" it could be that you no longer feel attractive towards your spouse and you want a new spark in your relationship, or you find it so hard carrying around the extra weight and with having your own kids young you want to be there for them with enough energy to play and have fun within these precious moments as you know they will not last forever.

You see where i am going here? So ask yourself through a few questions and starting writing down your answers. It may even surprise you when you dig deep what you come out with.

Now once you have your answers you can move onto the next step which is to keep those answers with you either all the time or somewhere you have quick access to so they are there for you instantly.

Why i say this is because when the times get tough and you have those bad days "which we all do", i need you to pick up the paper you have wrote your reasons why on, and use them for motivation to keep you back on track.

Finding your reason why can be a huge game changer for your lifestyle, so that's why it's so important to keep these personal reasons on hand.

The amount of people i see who don't write down there reasons why is extremely high, but what's even more crazy is the amount of people who don't even write down there goals!

To me this is madness... How do you know where you are going? If you haven't wrote down your body and lifestyle goals yet. So if you haven't, stop reading this part now and get writing!

But just before you do i need you to do one thing...

Make sure your goals are specific and clear. There's nothing worse than when i say to someone to see their goals and they show them to me which says, "i want to lose weight" or get into slimmer clothes.

My question is "how much weight" and "what size clothes" the more specific the better! It brings the goal more to life and more of a reality for you to personally relate to. Generic goals will give you generic results, and specific goals will give you specific results.

Write your goals out more like this example i will give you below...

"I will achieve my goal of weighing (fill in the number) by the date of (fill in the date)"

You see, you not only have a specific goal you want to achieve but you've also put a deadline on it, so you have to take action on it without slacking.

Now you have this goal setting tip along with "finding the reason why" and you can see why certain people will have better results than others because they have clearer action steps towards where they are heading.

Conclusion

Thank you again for downloading my book on Carb Cycling!

I hope this book will help you to lose your stubborn pounds, look great and feel amazing!

The next step is to make sure you take massive action on what I have taught you in this book.

Remember to use the success mindset principles which I gave you within the last section of this book. That will help you get started and stay on track!

Finally, if you enjoyed this book, then I'd like to ask you for a favor. Would you be kind enough to leave a review for this book on Amazon? It will be greatly appreciated!

Thank you and good luck!

Richard Huntley

P.S. Here's a list of healthy food groups you can bring into diet your through carb cycling:

Fat Burning Fruits

Strawberries

Pineapple

Blueberries

Blackberries

Cherries (my favourite)

Apples

Fat Burning Proteins

Turkey

Chicken

Beef

Salmon

Cod

Tuna

Eggs

Cottage Cheese

Fat Burning Carb Foods

White rice (basmati)

Potatoes

Shirataki Noodles

Buckwheat Pasta

Sprouted grain bread

Quinoa

Good Sources of Fat

Coconut oil

Avocado

Walnuts

Omega 3 eggs

Oily Fish

Olives

Flaxseed

Enclosing I thought it would be great to add a few chapters from my good friend and fellow author Kathy Hunt, with her bestselling "Anti-Inflammatory Diet" book.

Enjoy!

Anti-Inflammatory Diet

Beginners Guide To Avoid Inflammation and Eliminate Pain

By Kathy Hunt

Introduction

I want to welcome you to this amazing guide on the anti-inflammatory diet along with quick and easy recipes that you can make to help prevent and reduce your current inflammation.

Inside this book it contains proven steps and strategies on how to eliminate inflammation from your body to help ease pain and live and healthier, happier life.

You may want to read this short book over a few times to let the new knowledge sink in and enjoy the golden nuggets inside like so many other people have.

Let's dive right in!

Kathy Hunt

Chapter 1 – What is Inflammation?

Many of you must have read different medical opinions on what really is inflammation and certainly a lot of those reading these lines have tried to end up the pain with medication not that efficient as initially thought.

This is mainly because inflammation can be caused by various factors and is not always that most popular drugs can help.

Briefly, inflammation is a process by which some particular white cells of the body, also named leukocytes, together with substances they produce, have the function of protecting us from infection with foreign organisms, such as bacteria and viruses. Some individuals will think that this is normal and that inflammation is, therefore, a good sign. Acute inflammation prevents the spread of infectious agents and damage to nearby tissues, helps to remove damaged tissue and pathogens, and assists the body's repair processes.

There are situations in which, as studies proved, inflammation can lead to the development of degenerative diseases, and here we talk about chronic inflammation or silent inflammation, as Dr. Barry Sears, Ph.D. coined it.

This can be triggered by excessive calories consumption and oxidative stress. Stress-induced inflammation is strongly related to aging process.

Autoimmune response is yet another problem that inflammation could possibly represent. The body's defense system identifies an infection when, in fact, there are no foreign anti-corps that are invading the organism. The most common type of such physical affection is arthritis, which can be: rheumatoid, psoriatic or gouty.

Inflammation is able to produce a lot of symptoms which, remember, don't compulsory mean that you have somewhere in your body an inflammation.

From them we remind: redness, swollen joint that's sometimes warm to the touch, joint pain, joint stiffness, loss of joint function.

It can also be associated with general flu-like symptoms like for instance fever, chills, fatigue/loss of energy, headaches, loss of appetite, muscle stiffness.

However, you should notice that inflammation influences the health of your cardiovascular system, affects how quickly your injuries heal and plays a role in determining whether or not you catch a cold.

In order to determine if within your organism there has been settled an inflammation, you should take a blood test which measures two biomarkers linked to the presence of such: c-reactive protein and white blood cells.

C-reactive protein is directly related to the stage of inflammation, while white blood cells in great number don't necessarily prove that you have got an inflammation.

Their role is to fight infections, but their presence is also influenced by stress, trauma, allergies, certain diseases you could have.

Risk factors which increase the likelihood of developing chronic inflammation are closely related to age, obesity and diet, sexual hormones, smoking, sleep disorders, excessive blood glucose.

Studies connect a lot of types of affections with inflammation: allergy, Alzheimer's, anemia, Ankylosing Spondylitis, asthma, autism, arthritis, congestive heart failure, eczema, cardiovascular diseases, cancer, diabetes, macular degeneration (medical condition that usually affects older adults and results in a loss of vision in the center of the visual field, the macula, because of damage to the retina), chronic kidney disease, osteoporosis, depression, cognitive decline, pancreatitis, anemia, fibromyalgia, frailty, muscle wasting, fibrosis, heart attack, lupus, psoriasis, stroke.

It is proven that in some of these affections, inflammation is present in a certain shape, at cellular level or organ-directed level. Some of these are auto-immune diseases.

Cancer is terrifying and it can be connected to inflammation, but we have some good news: keeping under control inflammation can reduce chances that cancer develops. Chronic inflammation creates an ideal environment for free radicals, rogue molecules that travel through the body leaving a path of destruction in their wake. If a healthy cell's DNA is damaged by free radicals, it may mutate. Continuing to grow and divide, it may transform into a cancerous tumor. Therefore, free radicals stimulate the evolution of an inflammation.

Chapter 2 – Foods That Can Cause Inflammation

Not only can food increase the level of the inflammation, but it can add some more chronic conditions such as obesity, diabetes and heart disease.

Let's start with ingredients that can enhance your sufferance: white refined sugar, with the comment that natural carbohydrates are not damaging or saturated fat which can trigger fat tissue inflammation, contained in some kinds of cheese, meat, pasta and grain-based desserts, trans fats, encountered in fried products, processed snack foods, cookies, donuts, stick margarines, fast food.

To the list of substances that can trigger the body to produce pro-inflammatory chemicals we can add: omega 6 acids, found in oils such corn, safflower, sunflower, grape-seed, soy, peanut, refined carbohydrates composing white flour products, white rice, white potatoes, refined cereals products, mono-sodium glutamate , a flavor-enhancing food additive that can be found in soy sauce, different sorts of Asian food, prepared soups, salad dressings, deli meats, affecting the liver. Last, but not least, we should refrain from consuming products containing gluten and casein.

When you are trying to give up sugar in order to lose weight, have you reflected upon the effects the substitutes can have? Aspartame is a neurotoxin and if your body attacks it, then its response will be an inflammatory one.

Let's think about some wild party. Excessive use of alcohol disrupts multi-organ interactions and can cause inflammation.

For how many of you has the thought of being vegetarian or vegan become reality?

Well, you ought to know that meat and poultry tend to cause inflammation, but wild-caught fish can offer you omega 3, minerals and vitamins that protect your organism against chronic inflammation. With the purpose of counteracting inflammation, is important to balance the quantities of omega-3 and omega 6 acids that you ingest. We usually intake a surplus of omega-6 acids from sunflower or corn oil, which you can find in fast food and other processed products, as well as from oil-rich seeds.

Other enemies that contribute to this imbalanced ratio are margarine and partially hydrogenated vegetable oils. Oily fish, walnuts, flax, hemp, and to a lesser degree soy and sea vegetables, contain omega-3 acids.

Getting to the point, vegetarians, vegans or vegetarians that eat only fish as meat not only get more omega-3 acids, but more antioxidants in order to fight free-radicals that get to a high degree of inflammation.

Besides other products written above, dairy ones such as yoghurt, ice-cream, cottage cheese, butter, other kinds of cheese, are very often packed with hormones or antibiotics, so try to avoid them or at least try to identify from where they come and what is the trace of the product, the origin of ingredients and the manner in which the final product is obtained.

Iodized salt is sometimes depleted of its natural minerals with only sodium left or is refined using harmful substances as heavy metals or anti-caking additives that are not healthy.

Reading this gets you thinking that you will have to eliminate more than 50 percent of what you are usually eating? Don't worry, red meat, fat and carbohydrates are not so bad if they originate from natural, ecological or bio sources. Small producers still give attention to what they put in the food.

If you cannot afford them all the time, then at least you can be attentive to the way you mix different types of food when you consume them.

Substances and aliments proved to be efficient in curing and preventing inflammation-related diseases: ginger, melatonin, green leafs, resveratrol, vitamin D, zinc, magnesium, Gotu Kola – a herb, green tea, forest berries, papaya, turmeric, rosemary,

Sedentary lifestyle is another risk factor that can foster the development of chronic inflammation. Studies have shown that constant and not effort-exaggerated physical exercises can prevent diseases associated with it.

Bonus: Pick up a Free copy of my 7 Day Fat Loss Formula as a thank you for grabbing a copy of my carb cycling kindle book.

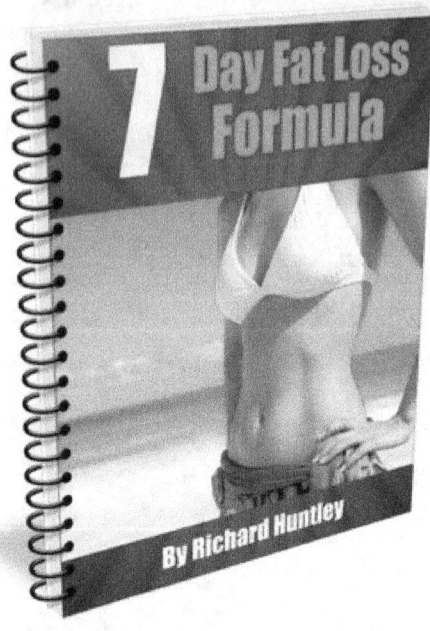

http://www.rhmartialfitness.com/freegift4u/kindle

Disclaimer

We urge all kindle readers to request medical or professional guidance before starting any weight loss plan, workout training regime or any diet. When participating on any new training plan we urge people to start slower and gradual.

This document is geared towards providing exact and reliable information in regards to the topic and issue covered. The publication is sold with the idea that the publisher is not required to render accounting, officially permitted, or otherwise, qualified services. If advice is necessary, legal or professional, a practiced individual in the profession should be ordered.

www.ingramcontent.com/pod-product-compliance
Lightning Source LLC
Chambersburg PA
CBHW060444290526
45793CB00002B/564